Seniors: We are Still Vital and Relevant

SENIORS:
We are Still Vital and Relevant

MARSHA NIXON POWELL

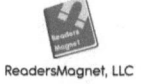

ReadersMagnet, LLC

Seniors: We are Still Vital and Relevant
Copyright © 2024 by Marsha Nixon Powell

Published in the United States of America

Library of Congress Control Number: 2024921624
ISBN   Paperback: 979-8-89091-715-7
ISBN   eBook: 979-8-89091-716-4

All rights reserved. No part of this publication may be reproduced, stored in a retrieval system or transmitted in any way by any means, electronic, mechanical, photocopy, recording or otherwise without the prior permission of the author except as provided by USA copyright law.

The opinions expressed by the author are not necessarily those of ReadersMagnet, LLC.

ReadersMagnet, LLC
10620 Treena Street, Suite 230 | San Diego, California, 92131 USA
1.619. 354. 2643 | www.readersmagnet.com

Book design copyright © 2024 by ReadersMagnet, LLC. All rights reserved.

Cover design by Jhiee Oraiz
Interior design by Dorothy Lee

TABLE OF CONTENTS

CHAPTER 1
We Are Appreciative 1

CHAPTER 2
Healthy Aging Tips 4

CHAPTER 3
Fun Things to Do - Games/Physical Activities 8

CHAPTER 4
Grandparenting 13

CHAPTER 5
Long Time Marriages/Loss of Loved Ones/Friends 20

CHAPTER 6
Staying Social 25

CHAPTER 7
Volunteering/Community Involvement 28

CHAPTER 8
Traveling Solo, But Not Necessarily Alone 32

CHAPTER 9
Independent Living/Living With Family Members 36

CHAPTER 10
Seniors: We Are Still Vital and Relevant 42

This book is dedicated to my family and in loving memory of my mother, Betty and my sister, Brenda.

ACKNOWLEDGMENTS

I would like to give love and appreciation to my daughters: Qiana and Cierra, and my grandson, Mark for their encouragement, and continued love and support.

CHAPTER 1
We Are Appreciative

Encouraging and uplifting words can have a profound impact on the well-being of senior citizens. As they face mental health concerns such as depression and anxiety, it becomes crucial to provide them with support and motivation through positive phrases and uplifting messages. While seniors have much to be grateful for, they may also struggle with feelings of loneliness, personal loss, and a loss of purpose. By engaging in regular communication and varying the forms of messages, including spoken words, notes, and cards, we can uplift their spirts and enhance their overall well-being.

The Importance of Encouragement for Seniors

As seniors navigate their golden years, they may experience feelings of loneliness, and loss, making encouragement an essential aspect of their lives.

If you have communication playing a vital role in providing encouragement to seniors, engaging in regular conversations that are motivational and inspiring can uplift their spirits and provide a sense of companionship. Active listening and using positive phrases for elderly people are key components of effective communication with seniors. In addition to verbal communication, personal words of encouragement can have a profound impact on the well-being of senior citizens. Expressions of love, asking how they are doing, and suggesting enjoyable activities are all ways to provide support and inspire seniors of their importance to make them feel valued, appreciated, and loved.

For seniors, gratitude is all about taking time to appreciate the here and now of our life's purpose and the responsibilities of each day.

What is Senior Appreciation?

Senior appreciation is more than just a concept. It's heartfelt expression of love, respect, and gratitude towards the other people in our lives. Our elders have a wealth of knowledge and life experiences that we can learn from. It can be accumulated wisdom and experience over the years, deserving of our utmost appreciation.

What are some ways to show appreciation for seniors?

Showing appreciation for seniors is a wonderful way to honor their wisdom and contributions. Here are some meaningful ways to express gratitude and make elders feel valued:

Ask them to teach you something. Ask questions, or seek advice. Whether it is baking, gardening, learning to sew, or cooking a beloved childhood meal.

Older people are a vital part of our society, but they are often overlooked. An encouraging word can help them realize we value them for their life experience and wisdom.

As they age, they may also face physical and emotional changes. This makes it easier for them to experience depression and hopelessness. When you offer words of encouragement it generates trust and confidence between people. In addition, it strengthens relationships and improves communication.

Seniors' contributions to society, their resilience, and their ability to guide and inspire younger generations are invaluable. Let us honor and celebrate our seniors for all they have done and continue to do.

"Age is an issue of mind over matter.
If you don't mind, it doesn't matter."
Mark Twain

CHAPTER 2
Healthy Aging Tips

As you age, maintaining good health becomes increasingly important. Here are some tips to help you stay healthy and age gracefully.

- Eat healthy. Maintaining a healthy diet as you age is essential for living well.
- Stay active – walk or physical activity on a regular basis.
- Make the most of your doctor check-ups doctor orders/ask questions if you don't understand something.
- Don't smoke
- Stay socially connected

Ten Habits That Age You

1. A constant diet of unhealthy foods
2. Consuming too much alcohol
3. Insufficient sleep
4. Overwhelming stress or anxiety
5. Too much time in the sun

6. A lack of activity or exercise
7. A smoking habit
8. Sitting too much
9. Not drinking enough water
10. High glucose levels

How you can improve your health as you get older.

As you age, there are several steps you can take to promote good health and maintain your well-being. Here are some practical steps:

1. Cardiovascular Health:

- Stay active: regular moderate physical activity, such as walking or swimming, helps maintain a healthy weight and lowers the risk of heart disease.
- Healthy diet: choose vegetables, fruits, whole grains, high-fiber foods, and lean protein sources (like fish). Limit saturated fat and salt intake.
- Avoid smoking: smoking contributes to artery hardening, high blood pressure, and increased heart rate. If you smoke, seek help to quit.

2. Bone, Joint, and Muscle Health:

- Calcium: consume adequate calcium from sources like dairy products, broccoli, kale, salmon and tofu.

- Strength and flexibility: engage in regular physical activity to maintain muscle strength, endurance, and flexibility. This helps with coordination, stability and balance.

3. General Health Tips:

- Stay active: keep your body and mind active. Regular physical activity is essential for overall health.
- Fall prevention: have your vision and hearing checked regularly. Remove clutter and fix loose rugs. Install handrails as needed.
- Regular Check-ups: talk to your doctor about health concerns you have.

Secrets for Aging Gracefully

- Eat a balanced diet
- Drink plenty of water – limit alcohol intake
- Consistent exercise
- Explore a sense of purpose
- Be strategic with skin and sun care

Remember, healthy aging involves a holistic approach that includes physical, mental, and social well-being. Incorporate these secrets into your lifestyle and you'll be on the path to aging gracefully.

Healthy living is healthy aging. Developing and maintaining healthy aging practices throughout the lifespan contributes to greater resilience and opportunities to thrive as we age – from infancy through older adulthood.

Small lifestyle changes can make a significant difference in your health as you grow older. Consult with your healthcare provider for personalized advice and recommendations.

> *"The older you get the more you realize you have no desire for drama, conflict or stress. You just want a cozy home, food on the table, and to be surrounded by kind people who make you happy."*
> *Anonymous*

CHAPTER 3
Fun Things to Do - Games/Physical Activities

When it comes to games for seniors (especially ones that stimulate the brain), there are so many options – Chess, Monopoly, Scrabble. Games are not only a form of childhood amusement. In fact, all senior citizens can reap the benefits of having fun.

Some of the best types of games and activities include:

- Active games and sports
- Dancing, Karaoke, and other performance arts
- Parties and other social gatherings
- Traditional games and puzzles
- Number games/word games – color by numbers, crossword/jig saw puzzles
- Group games for seniors – Bingo, Game Show games – "The Price is Right", "Family Feud", and "Wheel of Fortune", encourages large groups.

Games can be incredibly beneficial for seniors, providing not only entertainment, but also various cognitive and social advantages.

Key takeaways:

- Games provide opportunities for seniors to have fun, relieve stress, and exercise their brain.
- Puzzle, tile and board games offer mental challenges and opportunities for socializing.
- Video games provide visual and auditory engagements for seniors.
- Card games and dice games are convenient and portable options.
- Word games and outdoor games offer engaging activities for seniors.

Exercising for Seniors is a Good Idea

Staying physically active provides many health benefits. As you age, regular exercise can help you maintain better physical health, mental well-being, strength, flexibility, balance and an overall improved quality of life.

Some options include:

1. Balance Exercises

- One leg stance: stand behind a solid chair and hold on to the back for support. Lift one foot and balance on one leg. Repeat on the other leg.
- Heel-to-Toe Walk: stand beside a table or wall for support. Walk slowly, placing one foot in front of the other, touching the heel to the, toe.

2. Chair Exercises (perform 10-15 repetitions)

- Seated leg lifts
- Seated marching
- Seated knee extensions

Eight benefits of Chair Exercises: In addition to reducing fall risk, these chair exercises for seniors provide a host of other benefits.

They will help older adults:

11. Build and maintain muscle strength
12. Strengthen bones
13. Slow down osteoporosis
14. Keep joints, tendons, and ligaments more flexible
15. Improve coordination and flexibility
16. Increase energy
17. Strengthen heart and lungs
18. Promote greater sense of well-being

It's never too late to start exercising. Choose activities that you enjoy, and consult with a health care professional to tailor an exercise routine to your specific needs. Always remember to stay active and have fun!

8 Unique Activities for Seniors

1. Research your ancestry and make a family tree. There are numerous benefits for seniors who delve into their family's history, such as the increased sense awareness of self and identity it can bring about. It is also a great opportunity to form new relationships with cousins, aunts, uncles, etc. that one may have never known existed.

2. Start a blog. It gives people the opportunity to create stories about themselves and share them with other enthusiasts from around the world via blog posts written daily or whenever.

3. Become an umpire or referee. Sports are a great way to stay active, and they can also be a lot of fun.

4. Start quilting. Quilting is good for you. Not only does it help reduce stress and enhance creativity, quilt clubs provide an opportunity to socialize with other members.

5. Learn an instrument. Music is an excellent way to keep the mind active and engaged. There are so many instruments that will fit any interest or skill level. For example, drumming or learning to play the guitar.

6. Find your long-lost friends. Catching up with old friends is always a good time, and social media makes it easy.

7. Enjoy birdwatching. Birds are fascinating creatures that provide an excellent source of entertainment and education. This is a great way to get outdoors, learn about nature from observing our feathered friends in their natural habitats all around you.

8. Taking a boat ride on the lake. There is nothing like a peaceful boat ride on a calm lake to soothe the soul. Taking a boat ride is the perfect activity to relax and enjoy nature.

CHAPTER 4
Grandparenting

How to be a Better Grandparent

Grandparenting is an opportunity to play, to love someone new, to appreciate the magic of a developing mind, and to be needed by someone again.

Grandparents can:

- Share the world in a new way through younger eyes.

- Share the things they're passionate about with a new audience.

- Provide input that parents cannot.

- Watch children develop through all stages of growth.

- Provide expanded support and encouragement to their grandchildren.

The Role of a Grandparent in a Child's Life

- Grandparents can play different roles, depending on the family configuration and needs. Some grandparenting requires full-time commitment. For others, grandparents may fix meals and provide financial support to their grandchildren. However, grandparenting can go beyond these material contributions from words of wisdom, or emotional support. For others, grandparenting is a weekend together, an afternoon play date, summer vacation, a chat on the phone, or a text or email exchange every now and then.

- A good first step to a long and successful relationship with your grandchild is to establish ground rules with their parents. Be clear about what role you want to have in your grandchild's life. Let them know how often you want to babysit, for example, or whether you'd like to be included in events such as school functions.

- Talk with parents about their rules. Consistency is important for kids, know the behavior limits your grandchild has to follow at home and maintain those rules when they are with you.

- Babyproof your home to ensure safety for infants and toddlers since it's probably been a number of years since you had young children in your home. Check with grandchild's parents about ways to babyproof your home, so they're comfortable leaving the child with you.

- Enforce any agreed upon punishment for bad behavior, whether it's a "time out" or loss of privileges, for example.

Common grandparenting pitfalls to avoid:

To avoid potential conflict within your family, try to avoid these common grandparenting pitfalls:

- Trying to be the parent. As much as you might want to tell your children how to raise your grandkids, it is not your role. Respect the parenting decisions your children make for your grandkids.

- Buying your grandkid's affection. It is tempting for grandparents to shower their grandchildren with gifts, but check with the child's parents before you buy more toys. Maybe substitute some of your gift giving with activities instead. Do something with your grandchild that you both love and will build memories. Shower them with love instead of gifts.

- Overindulging the first few grandchildren and then being able to repeat it as additional grandchildren come along. This can cause resentment from your own children who have kids later in life. Remember, that whatever you do for your first grandchild (college fund, beach vacations, trip to the zoo, etc.) will set a precedent that you might feel pressured for every other grandchild.

Making the Most of Your Grandparenting Time

- Carve out one-on-one time. On occasion, spend time with individual grandchildren. It will give you an opportunity to bond, without competition. One grandchild at a time.

- See the sights. Concerts and plays, movies, science centers and museums, parks, or walks in the neighborhood provide opportunities to be together and to exchange ideas and opinions.

Life Lessons from Grandparents

Grandparents can teach you many lessons that help to answer the great questions of life. It's wisdom that doesn't go out of fashion, and which the passing years only confirms. Grandparents, with their vast experience of mind and heart, become true mentors who show us a unique perspective on things.

When we were growing up, we didn't have access to information or resources as easily as the young people have today, and yet we learned countless lessons. We've faced hard times, often including wars and other crises. We've run companies and raised families, and our work hasn't always been recognized.

12 Reasons Why Grandparents Are Key to a Child's Happiness

1. Unconditional love and support. Grandparents provide unwavering love and support to grandchildren, creating a nurturing environment filled with warmth, love and reassurance.

2. Family history and heritage. Grandparents are the storytellers of family history, passing down traditions and cultural heritage to grandchildren.

3. Wisdom and life lessons. Grandparents are repositories of life's wisdom, offering invaluable guidance and lessons gleaned from decades of experience.

4. Role models and resilience. Grandparents demonstrate strength and perseverance in facing life's challenges. Through their own experiences, they teach grandchildren invaluable wisdom about overcoming adversity and bouncing back from setbacks.

5. Spoiling with affection. Grandparents have a knack for showering grandchildren with affection, gestures, and treats, often indulging them in ways that parents might not.

6. Supporting parents. Grandparents are a crucial support system for parents, helping with childcare responsibilities and household tasks.

7. Teaching life skills. Grandparents are invaluable teachers of practical life skills, imparting knowledge that extends beyond the classroom.

8. Grandparents are instrumental in celebrating the milestones of a child's life. Whether it's a birthday, graduation, or extraordinary achievement, grandparents are essential in creating meaningful and joyous experiences for grandchildren.

9. Building confidence. Grandparents are champions of confidence-building, offering unwavering support and encouragement that bolsters a child's self-assurance.

10. Nurturing creativity. Grandparents nurture creativity in grandchildren through various activities like story-

telling, arts and crafts, and imaginative play.

11. Cultural enrichment. Grandparents are cultural ambassadors, introducing grandchildren to customs, languages, and traditions.

12. Legacy of love. Grandparents' affectionate presence creates a nurturing environment where children flourish emotionally, which imprints a profound sense of belonging and security in grandchildren's hearts, fostering bonds that withstand the test of time.

"When parents turn into grandparents, something magical happens." - unknown

CHAPTER 5
Long Time Marriages/ Loss of Loved Ones/Friends

Late-life marriages among seniors are becoming increasingly common as people live longer, it is more normative to remarry after being widowed or divorced.

If a second marriage ends in divorce, as long as it lasted 10 years or longer, you can choose between the two spouses' benefits.

Long-time Marriages Among Seniors:

- Many older adults remained in their marriages for a long period of time.

- At least half of those who married in the 1970s reached their 25th anniversary.

- At least 59% of adults ages 60 and older have been married just once.

- Among those ages 60 to 69, 46% of men and 39% of women are still married to the first and only person they wed.

How To Celebrate Anniversaries:

Celebrating anniversaries is a wonderful way to honor and cherish the time you've spent together with your partner. Whether it's your wedding anniversary, the date you met, or any other significant milestone, where you have thoughtful ideas to make the occasion special:

- Romantic Dinner: plan a candlelight dinner at home or at a favorite restaurant. Choose a menu that holds sentimental value or try a new cuisine together.

- Recreate your first date: take a trip down memory lane by revisiting the place where you had your first date. Reminisce about the special day and create new memories.

- Weekend Getaway: escape for a weekend to a cozy bed-and-breakfast, a beachside cottage, or a scenic cabin. Disconnect from daily life and focus on each other.

- Renew Your Vows: if you're celebrating a significant anniversary (like 10, 25 or 50 years), consider renewing your wedding vows. Invite close friends and family to witness your special moment.

- Watch your wedding video or look through your wedding album: relive the magic of your wedding day by watching your wedding video or looking through old photo albums, share stories and laughter as you reminisce.

- Plan a surprise date: surprise your partner with a fun activity they've always wanted to do. It could be a hot air balloon ride, a dance class, or a scenic hike.

Remember, the most meaningful celebrations come from the heart. Tailor your anniversary celebration to your unique relationship, and enjoy the love you share.

How Many Older Couples Live Together Outside of Marriage?

The number of adults older than 50 who were living together outside of marriage more than doubled between 2000 and 2010, from 1.2 million to 2.75 million, according to the Journal of Marriage and Family.

Widowhood

Widowhood is particularly common among older women compared to older men due to differences – life experiences. Women on an average live longer than men. Among those 75 years or older who have ever married, 58% of women and 28% of men had experienced the death of a spouse in their lifetime, making this stage of life particularly difficult for older adults. The proportion of those who are currently widowed is relatively lower than for those widowed at one point because some respondents who lost a spouse eventually remarried becoming "currently married" instead of "currently widowed."

Coping With Grief

The effects of losing a loved one can include:

- Emotional Changes: people might feel or act differently than usual.

- Physical Health Impact: grief can be exhausting and weaken the immune system.

- Spiritual Experiences: some may have dreams about their loved one.

- Complicated Grief and Depression: These can be complications of mourning.

Coping with the loss of a close friend or family member may be one of the hardest challenges that many of us face when we lose a spouse, sibling, or parent, our grief can be particularly intense. Human beings are naturally resilient, considering most of us can endure loss and then continue on with our lives, but some people feel unable to carry out daily activities. Individuals with severe grief may benefit from the help of a psychologist or another licensed mental health professional with a specialization in grief. Remember and celebrate the lives of your loved ones. Honor a loved one by collecting donations to a favorite charity of the deceased, passing on a family name to a baby, or plant a garden in their memory.

The Grief of Losing a Loved One

Whether it's a close friend, spouse, partner, parent, sibling, child, or other relative, few things are as painful as losing someone you love. After such a significant loss, life may never seem quite the same again. But in time, you can ease your sorrow, start to look to the future, and eventually come to terms with your loss.

> *"The loss of a loved one doesn't mean they are gone. Their spirit still lives within us."*
> *Kately Spotten*

CHAPTER 6
Staying Social

Seniors who socialize regularly are less likely to experience feelings of despair and worthiness. Mental health has a significant impact on a person's wellness as well as their outlook on life in a retirement community because of the benefits of social interactions.

Eight Reasons Why Seniors Need to Have a Social Life:

1. Having an active social life encourages better mental health. It helps lower the risk of depression, and also prevents feelings of isolation.

2. Socializing encourages seniors to be physically active. Seniors who are social, getting out and meeting people, have a profound effect on their overall health. Physical activity reduces the risk of illnesses.

3. Social activities give seniors a sense of belonging. Socializing helps elderly adults feel they have a place where they belong which allows them to connect with peers or strengthen bonds with younger generations.

4. Socializing with friends help seniors lower stress and improve their mood.

5. Socialization can boost a seniors self-worth. Friends and loved ones make us feel better about ourselves. Everyone deserves to feel worthy of living. The people around us remind us of what makes us unique and valuable. This gives us meaning in our lives. Friendship requires give and take. Being a part of that makes a person understand that they are needed and wanted.

6. Seniors can socialize for increased cognitive function. They tend to perform better on related tests compared to those who have less interaction with close partners.

7. Social interactions inspire positive living. Older adults who share strong friendships tend to have a more positive outlook. They are usually happier and experience a better quality of life compared to those who are isolated.

8. Socially active seniors tend to live longer. Current data has shown that a varied social circle helps many seniors. This is primarily because of the many other benefits that come with being socially active.

How To Stay Social as You Age

- Reconnect with friends and family
- Learn a new skill or language
- Embrace technology – take an online class
- Give to others – volunteer to have a purpose and feel part of a community

Final Thoughts

People change throughout their lifetimes, and that is especially true in the older years.

By encouraging older adults to participate in social activities and fostering a supportive environment, we can then maintain a vibrant fulfilling life. But no matter what, everyone needs to be around people.

"Count your age by friends, not years,
Count your life by smiles not tears."
John Lennon

CHAPTER 7
Volunteering/Community Involvement

Volunteering as a senior is not just a way to spend time but also a chance to grow, connect with the community and find personal satisfaction. You can make a difference by helping at a local food bank, guiding/tutoring young people, or assisting at a community garden. Such activities give you a sense of purpose and can make you feel good.

6 Benefits of Volunteering for Older Adults

1. It's good for mental health. Volunteering keeps the brain active, which contributes to good mental health. Meaningful and productive activities can help you feel happier and have a positive outlook on life.

2. It prevents loneliness and isolation. Social isolation is a major issue that many seniors face. The feeling of loneliness and few interactions with others can negatively impact a person's health. Getting out into the community and volunteering promotes socialization.

3. It gives you a feeling of purpose. Regaining a feeling of purpose through volunteering can

help older adults feel recharged with a new zest for life. It can also be a motivating factor for setting and accomplishing other goals.

4. It helps you meet new friends. Volunteering is a great way to meet new people with common interest. By working together towards the same mission, you can build friendships with like-minded peers who are finding creative solutions in your community.

5. Volunteering for older adults increases physical activity. Physical activity is highly important when it comes to staying healthy and independent as we age. Volunteering keeps you moving whether you are serving meals at a shelter, helping to clean up your local parks, or walking around the neighborhood, with someone as a companion.

6. It helps you learn new skills. Many volunteer activities allow you to try things you've never done before and learn new skills. Take a chance at opportunities that are a little outside of your comfort zone. You may develop a passion you never knew you had.

Community Involvement

Community Involvement allows seniors to connect with the community, engage with different groups, and contribute to community development. This involvement can lead to stronger community ties and a sense of belonging.

Seniors can stay involved in their communities by:

- Participating in Cooking Demonstrations: many senior living communities organize cooking demonstrations where residents can learn new recipes, socialize, and enjoy delicious food.

- Attending Live Concerts/Dance Parties: music has a powerful impact on emotions and well-being. Attending live concerts within the community allows seniors to enjoy music and to dance together.

- Joining Group Exercise Classes: participating in group exercise classes promotes physical fitness and offers mental and emotional benefits.

- Participate in Local Events and Clubs: Board games – seniors can join local board games groups or organize game meetings with friends. Board games enhance cognitive skills and provide social interaction.

- Join Arts and Crafts Workshops: seniors can explore their creative side by participating in art classes or craft workshops.

- Books Clubs for Seniors:

- Offers a way to stay mentally active and socially engaged

- Can be organized by gathering a group of interested individuals

- Joining book clubs fosters a love for reading and creates a sense of community that incorporates discussion questions and activities

> *"The health benefits of volunteerism and community involvement are well documented including its impact on increasing longevity. It is even more powerful when your efforts give you a sense of purpose in life."* – Bryan James, an epidemiologist at the Rush Alzheimer's Disease Center – Chicago, Illinois

CHAPTER 8
Traveling Solo, But Not Necessarily Alone

Traveling can be a wonderful way for seniors to experience new environments. Joining a senior travel group can help explore new destinations while ensuring safety and accommodating specific needs. Travel groups also provide a social setting to meet others who share a sense of adventure whether it's a cruise, a guided tour, or a simple road trip. Travel can broaden your horizons and provide fresh topics for conversation.

Traveling solo, but not alone. Celebrate a Solo Tour. Experience the thrill and independence of traveling on your own, with a Tour Director and with 24/7 support. Plus, curated activities for bonding with new friends.

Solo doesn't have to mean alone. Solo Tours are specifically for solo travelers, with plenty of time to explore on your own and other one-of-a-kind perks.

Why guided solo travel for seniors is a great adventure to try:

- You'll be part of a close-knit community. Everyone on your tour will be solo too. You can explore alongside other travelers who share your curiosity about the world and their craving for meaningful connections.

- You'll bond over exclusive experiences. Get to know your fellow solo travelers on a sunset cruise, in a cooking class, or through a restorative yoga class, unique exhilarating and mouthwatering group activities are included with your trip.

Is it safe for older women to travel alone?

Nearly 40% of older women (8.1 million) live alone. Living alone can foster a sense of independence, but it can also raise health and safety risks. It is important for women who live alone to stay socially active by keeping in touch with friends and family in person and online.

Solo travel for seniors can be a fantastic idea, offering independence, adventure, and the chance to explore the world at your own pace. Here are some considerations and tips to make when thinking about solo adventures:

1. Safety and plan:

- Choose safe destinations: opt for destinations with low crime rates and have healthcare facilities.

- Research local customs: understand local customs, safety tips, and any specific considerations for seniors.

- Stay connected: keep in touch with families and friends during your trip.

2. Group Tours:

- Small Group Tours: consider joining small groups designed for solo travelers. These tours provide companionship and expert local guides.

- Explore with like-minded travelers: joining a group allows you to share experiences with other adventure lovers.

3. Trip Options:

- Walking Vacations: Walk the World: Offers walking and hiking tours for travelers over 50 who want to be immersed in their chosen destinations.

- Guided Walking Tours: A secure and entertaining way for elderly individuals to discover new places.

- Cycling Tours: If you love cycling, consider group cycling tours that explore scenic landscapes without challenging terrains.

- Discovery Trips: Fully guided trips to Southeast Asia, Africa, or other regions can be exciting for solo travelers.

4. Embrace Independence:

- Solo travel allows you to wander freely, discover hidden gems, and create your itinerary.
- Trust your instincts, avoid risky situations, and have a backup plan for emergencies.

Remember, solo travel can be an enriching experience at any stage of life!

For more information and practical advice, check out the comprehensive guide on Solo Senior Travel. If you're ready to explore, consider joining one of the senior singles tours.

CHAPTER 9
Independent Living/Living With Family Members

Independent Living - Seniors living independently are older adults who are able to do daily activities without assistance. They live in housing arrangements designed exclusively for them, such as apartments, condos or houses. These settings offer meals, services, activities and social gatherings that make life easier and more enjoyable for residents. Some independent living communities may also provide health care services on-site or on-call.

Independent Senior Living Communities are great for aging adults who want to stay engaged socially while having a place that truly feels like home.

What is Independent Living?

Independent Living is any housing arrangement designed exclusively for older adults, generally 55 and over. Housing varies widely, from apartment-style living to single-family detached homes. The housing is friendlier to aging adults, often being more compact, with easier navigation and no maintenance or yardwork to worry about.

Since independent living facilities are aimed at older adults who need little or no assistance with activities of daily living (ADL), most do not offer medical or nursing staff. You can, however, hire in-home help separately as required.

As with any change in living situation, it is important to plan ahead and give yourself time and space to cope with change. By using these tips, you can find an independent living arrangement that makes your life easier, prolongs your independence, and enables you to thrive in your retirement.

There are many types of independent living facilities, from apartment complexes to stand-alone houses, which range in cost and services provided.

Tips for making the transition to independent living easier.

In addition to adjusting to a new living environment, you'll be meeting new neighbors and probably being introduced to new activities. You may feel stressful in the beginning, but there are things to do to make the transition easier:

- Decorate your new home. Hang familiar pictures, paint the walls, and make sure you have space for your most important possessions – a favorite armchair or treasured bookcase.

- Pack well in advance of the move. Don't add to the stress of the actual move by putting yourself in a position where you'll need to make hasty decisions about what to take and what to discard.

- Know what to expect. Do your homework on the independent living facility and make sure all of your questions are answered ahead of time. It will be less stressful if you know what to expect.

- Socialize. You may be tempted to stay in your apartment or house, but you'll feel comfortable much quicker if you get out there to meet the other residents, participate in activities, and explore the amenities.

To help decide if independent living is the right choice for you, answer the following four questions:

1. How easy is it for you to maintain your current house? Maintaining a home may be a longstanding source of pride for you, but it can also become a burden as you age. Perhaps your home has a large yard which requires constant maintenance, or increased crime may mean that your neighborhood is now too dangerous to walk around safely. Some of these challenges may be partially remedied by hiring outside help. However, as you'd like a place that does not require a lot of maintenance or worry, independent living may give

you more freedom and flexibility in the long run.

2. Is it difficult for you to connect to friends and family? The more isolated you are, the greater your risk for depression and other mental health problems. Independent living facilities can give you a built-in social network of peers, while many also provide structured activities, such as sports, arts, or field trips.

3. How easy is it for you to get around? You may live in an area where you have to drive to attend social activities, visit friends, and shop. If you find yourself less comfortable with driving, you may find yourself relying more and more on public transportation or family and friends to get around. It may be harder to visit others, pursue activities you enjoy, or keep doctor's appointments.

4. How is your health (and the health of your spouse)? It is important to consider your current and future health. For example, if you have a health condition that makes it difficult to stay active and will most likely worsen with time, it is good to consider your options carefully. It is

also important to consider the health of your spouse if you are married. Can you manage the activities of daily living, such as washing, showering, eating? Can you manage your finances? Can you manage medications and doctor appointments? If you are needing only minor assistance with activities of daily living, independent living may be right for you.

Considering Living with Family? Here are the Pros and Cons.

Seniors facing health or financial challenges may consider the option of moving with family. For seniors no longer able to live independently or who find assisted living too expensive, moving in with adult children or other relatives becomes a serious consideration.

Pros and Cons of living with family:

A senior moving in with family brings the stability to share in household expenses, such as mortgage payments, rent, utilities, and many times seniors are healthy enough to assist with childcare and provide valuable mentoring. But as seniors age, families find a need to bring in outside help on an occasional basis or event, 24-hour care to deal with family issues that arise. Having a senior move in also can create relationship issues if care-giving is needed. Of course, it also provides an opportunity for them to connect with their children and grandchildren.

As seniors age, health care demands also play a greater role in daily living. Some families may not have the skill or patience to deal with those needs. The rise of dementia and Alzheimer's can put many family relationships to the test.

The Bottom Line

Living with others offers a way to stay independent and avoid a cascade of mental, emotional, and physical health problems.

Isolation and loneliness are risk factors for many health problems. "When you live alone, you're at a higher risk for memory decline, depression, heart disease, diabetes, arthritis, and stress." Says Dr. Stevens, Stamford Medicine. "But having someone in the home is socially and mentally stimulating and it may help prevent health problems."

CHAPTER 10
Seniors: We Are Still Vital and Relevant

How You Can Remain Vital and Relevant as You Get Older

Becoming less relevant is one aspect of aging that can catch us by surprise. It sneaks up on us. One day we have purpose and then we feel it slipping away. We retire and our work colleagues get along just fine without us. We raise our children and they grow up and no longer need us.

Steps We Can Take to Maintain Our Relevance

1. Team up with Millennials instead of seeing them as a threat. Both sides have something to teach and learn from each other.

2. Don't resist change just because it's different. Be open to new ideas, even if that means letting go of the ways things have always been.

3. Keep up to date on learning new skills and the many ways we can be available to learn them.

4. Establish your own personal branding and market yourself and your skills.

5. Networking is still important, but it's a two-way street. Don't forget to ask how you can help those you need.

6. Think more like an entrepreneur, by being a perpetual learner and accountable for building your own business life. Don't rely on an organization to take care of you.

The Vital Connection: Seniors and Healthcare

As you journey through life, our healthcare needs evolve as we enter our golden years. For seniors, healthcare isn't just about ailments; it is about preserving independence, maintaining vitality, and enhancing quality of life.

Regular healthcare check-ups and screenings are essential for seniors to monitor their health and detect any potential issues early on from blood pressure issues to cancer screenings. These preventive measures can make all the difference in managing conditions before they escalate.

Moreover, managing chronic conditions becomes increasingly crucial with age. Whether its diabetes, arthritis, or heart disease, seniors must work closely with healthcare professionals to develop personalized treatment plans and adopt life-style modifications that promote well-being.

Mental health also plays a significant role in overall wellness for seniors. Combatting loneliness, staying socially engaged, and seeking support needed are vital aspects of maintaining emotional well-being.

In navigating the healthcare landscape, seniors should feel empowered to ask questions, seek clarification, and advocate for their needs. Building strong relationships with healthcare providers fosters trust and ensure that seniors receive the personalized care they deserve.

By prioritizing preventing care, managing chronic conditions, and nurturing well-being, seniors can navigate their healthcare journey with confidence and resilience, which will help you to remain vital and relevant during your senior years.

Here Are a Few Lessons That Can Be Learned from Seniors

- Embrace family traditions and build a home for everyone.

- Take care of your mind by reading. Reading can give you strength, comfort and healing.

- Don't stop learning and bringing yourself up to date. You can attend monthly educational classes or take classes online.

- Stay active. You'll never too old to do things and to have a rich and active social life.

- Enjoy a good conversation. Share life experiences with others and don't skimp on having friends of all ages, beliefs, cultures and social classes.

Ageless Icons: Eight Celebrities Who Are Baby Boomers:

1. Diane Keaton, 78. Her acting career has spanned five decades with no sign of slowing down.

2. Steven Spielberg, born in 1946. Spielberg was the producer, screenwriter, and director of box office blockbusters like Jaws, Close Encounter of the Third Kind, and the first three Indiana Jones movies.

3. Cher, 78. Her entertainment career started a half of the musical group Sonny & Cher. She then turned to acting, garnering critical acclaim for her roles in Silkwood and Mask.

4. Samuel L. Jackson is one of Hollywood's most bankable actors, with several decades in his acting career. Born in 1948, he started his acting career performing on stage.

5. Tom Hanks, born in 1956. He is considered by many to be a natural treasure, Academy Award winner. Tom

Hanks is one of the most beloved actors in Hollywood.

6. Tom Cruise, born in 1962. Tom Cruise's acting career took off in the 1980s with his box office hit Risky Business. His performances in such films as Rain Man, Top Gun, and Jerry Maguire secured his place as one of Hollywood's leading men.

7. George Clooney, born in 1961. Clooney is an actor and director, and starred in the Ocean Eleven's franchises.

8. Sandra Bullock. Born in 1964, started her career on the stage with minor roles and then moved on to becoming a household name when she starred in Speed.

We Are Always Relevant

Even if only for ourselves, we never really lose our relevance. Maybe no one's looking for us to lead the next project, but our grandkids might think we are the greatest thing since sliced bread. We'll always have value from those who love and care for us.

So, instead of looking back to see what we've lost, let's look to what we've gained.

Because when we're not being driven to prove to the world how much we still matter, we can let go and just engage with those who matter to us now.

"It Gets Greater Later" – Bevy Smith

ABOUT THE AUTHOR

Marsha Nixon Powell is a Philadelphia native. She lives with her family in Northeast Philadelphia. She is a long-time cancer survivor, who has been a business owner, and currently works as a Behavioral Health Technician in the Philadelphia School system with autistic and special-needs students.

She also works as a Home Caregiver for Senior Citizens in the Philadelphia and Bucks County areas. She is an inspiration to those who know her and continues to learn and develop new leadership and professional skills. She recently wrote her second book – ***The Many Rewards and Challenges of Being a Caregiver***.

Marsha is a hard worker, and in spite of her many ailments and chronic conditions, she is still going strong at seventy-four years of age!

www.ingramcontent.com/pod-product-compliance
Lightning Source LLC
LaVergne TN
LVHW041553070526
838199LV00046B/1938